EAT TO BEAT IBS

The Irritable Bowel Syndrome Diet: A Comprehensive Guide To Restoring Digestive Harmony

DR. LONDYN DELANEY

Table of Contents

Introductory

Irritable Bowel Syndrome; abbreviated as IBS. The large intestine (colon) is the typical target of this prevalent gastrointestinal illness. Symptoms of irritable bowel syndrome (IBS) include nausea, vomiting, cramps, bloating, gas, constipation, and abdominal discomfort.

Although the precise etiology of irritable bowel syndrome remains unknown, dietary variables, stress, hormones, and gut flora imbalances are all potential contributors. The impact on quality of life can be substantial due to the chronic nature of irritable bowel syndrome (IBS), the severity of which can vary from person to person.

The primary goal of treatment is symptom management, which can be achieved through a combination of medication, dietary changes, stress management techniques, and, in some cases, counseling or therapy to address underlying psychological issues.

CHAPTER ONE
Understanding Ibs Symptoms

Irritable Bowel Syndrome (IBS) presents a variety of symptoms, which can vary widely among individuals. The primary symptoms include:

• **Abdominal Pain and Cramping**: Often the most common symptom, this pain is typically felt in the lower abdomen and is relieved after a bowel movement.

• **Bloating and Gas**: Many people with IBS experience bloating, which can cause discomfort and a feeling of fullness.

• **Diarrhea (IBS-D)**: Some people with IBS predominantly experience diarrhea, characterized by frequent, loose, or watery stools.

- **Constipation (IBS-C)**: Others may experience constipation, with infrequent, hard, or lumpy stools.

- **Alternating Bowel Habits (IBS-M)**: Some individuals alternate between periods of diarrhea and constipation.

- **Mucus in Stool**: Presence of white mucus in the stool is a symptom that some people with IBS experience.

- **Urgent Need to Defecate**: There may be a sudden, strong urge to have a bowel movement, which can be difficult to control.

- **Incomplete Evacuation**: Feeling that a bowel movement is incomplete, even after going to the bathroom.

Triggers And Aggravating Factors

Certain factors can trigger or worsen IBS symptoms, including:

• **Food**: Specific foods and drinks (like dairy products, alcohol, caffeine, fatty foods, and some fruits and vegetables) can trigger symptoms in some people.

• **Stress**: Emotional stress can exacerbate symptoms.

• **Hormones**: Women may find that symptoms are worse during their menstrual periods, suggesting a hormonal link.

Diagnosis And Management

IBS is diagnosed based on symptoms and by ruling out other conditions. There is no specific test for IBS, but doctors may perform tests to exclude other diseases, such as celiac disease or inflammatory bowel disease.

Management of IBS often involves:

• **Dietary Changes**: Identifying and avoiding trigger foods, eating high-fiber foods, and sometimes following a low-FODMAP diet.

• **Medications**: Depending on symptoms, doctors might prescribe fiber supplements, laxatives, anti-diarrheal medications, antispasmodics, or antidepressants.

• **Lifestyle Changes**: Regular exercise, adequate sleep, and stress management techniques like mindfulness, yoga, or cognitive-behavioral therapy (CBT).

When To See A Doctor

It's important to consult a healthcare provider if you experience severe or persistent symptoms, significant weight loss, rectal bleeding, or symptoms that do not improve with initial treatment. These may indicate a more serious condition that requires medical evaluation.

Importance Of Diet In Managing IBS

Diet plays a crucial role in managing Irritable Bowel Syndrome (IBS) and can significantly impact the severity and frequency of symptoms. Here are some key points about the importance of diet in managing IBS:

Identifying Trigger Foods

Certain foods and drinks can trigger or worsen IBS symptoms. Common triggers include:

- **Dairy Products**: Lactose intolerance can exacerbate symptoms.
- **Gluten**: Some people with IBS may have non-celiac gluten sensitivity.
- **FODMAPs**: These are fermentable oligosaccharides, disaccharides, monosaccharides, and polyols that can cause bloating and gas.
- **Fatty Foods**: High-fat foods can trigger symptoms in some people.

- **Caffeine and Alcohol**: These can stimulate the intestines and worsen symptoms.

- **Artificial Sweeteners**: Sugar substitutes like sorbitol and mannitol can cause digestive issues.

Low-FODMAP Diet:

The low-FODMAP diet is specifically designed to reduce the intake of certain carbohydrates that are poorly absorbed in the small intestine. It involves three phases:

- **Elimination**: Avoiding all high-FODMAP foods for a few weeks.

- **Reintroduction**: Gradually reintroducing high-FODMAP foods one at a time to identify specific triggers.

- **Personalization**: Developing a long-term eating plan based on individual tolerance.

High-Fiber Diet:

For those with IBS-C (constipation-predominant IBS), increasing fiber intake can help. However, it's important to:

- **Choose Soluble Fiber**: Foods like oats, barley, and apples are gentler on the digestive system compared to insoluble fiber found in whole grains and vegetables.
- **Gradually Increase Fiber**: To avoid worsening symptoms, fiber intake should be increased gradually.

Regular Meal Patterns:

Eating regular, balanced meals can help manage symptoms. Tips include:

- **Small, Frequent Meals**: Eating smaller meals more frequently can reduce the load on the digestive system.

- **Avoiding Large Meals**: Large meals can cause bloating and discomfort.

- **Staying Hydrated**: Drinking plenty of water helps with digestion, especially when increasing fiber intake.

Specific Dietary Adjustments:

- **Probiotics**: These can help balance gut bacteria and improve symptoms for some people.

- **Peppermint Oil**: Known for its antispasmodic properties, it can help reduce abdominal pain and cramping.

- **Avoiding Gas-Producing Foods**: Foods like beans, lentils, carbonated drinks, and certain vegetables (e.g., broccoli, cauliflower) can increase gas and bloating.

IBS affects individuals differently, so it's important to develop a personalized dietary plan. Working with a healthcare provider or a registered dietitian can help identify specific dietary triggers and create an effective management plan tailored to individual needs.

Keeping a food diary to track what you eat and how it affects your symptoms can be very helpful. Regularly reviewing and adjusting your diet based on these observations can lead to better management of IBS symptoms over time.

Diet is a cornerstone of managing IBS. Identifying and avoiding trigger foods, adopting a low-FODMAP diet if necessary, ensuring adequate fiber intake, and maintaining regular meal patterns can all contribute to reducing symptoms and improving quality of life for individuals with IBS.

CHAPTER TWO
Common Triggers And Causes

IBS (Irritable Bowel Syndrome) can be influenced by a variety of triggers and underlying causes. Understanding these can help in managing and alleviating symptoms. Here are some common triggers and potential causes:

Common Triggers

Food and Diet:

• **High-FODMAP Foods**: Foods high in fermentable oligosaccharides, disaccharides, monosaccharides, and polyols (e.g., certain fruits, vegetables, grains, and dairy products) can exacerbate symptoms.

• **Dairy Products**: Lactose intolerance can cause digestive issues in some people with IBS.

• **Gluten**: Some individuals may have non-celiac gluten sensitivity.

• **Fatty Foods**: High-fat foods can trigger IBS symptoms.

• **Caffeine and Alcohol**: Both can irritate the digestive system.

• **Artificial Sweeteners**: Substitutes like sorbitol and mannitol can cause bloating and diarrhea.

Stress:

• **Emotional Stress**: Stress can affect the gut-brain axis, exacerbating IBS symptoms.

• **Psychological Factors**: Anxiety and depression are often linked to IBS, as stress can increase intestinal sensitivity and motility.

Hormonal Changes:

• **Menstrual Cycle**: Hormonal fluctuations during menstruation can worsen IBS symptoms in women.

Medications:

• **Antibiotics**: These can disrupt the gut microbiome, potentially triggering IBS symptoms.

• **Certain Painkillers**: Opioids and NSAIDs can affect bowel function.

Illness:

- **Gastrointestinal Infections**: A history of severe infection can lead to post-infectious IBS.

Potential Causes

Abnormal Gut Motility:

- **Altered Bowel Movement**: IBS can involve changes in the speed of digestion, leading to diarrhea or constipation.

Visceral Hypersensitivity:

- **Increased Sensitivity**: People with IBS often have a heightened sensitivity to abdominal pain and discomfort.

Gut-Brain Interaction:

• **Gut-Brain Axis**: Dysregulation between the brain and the gastrointestinal tract can contribute to IBS symptoms.

Microbiome Imbalance:

• **Gut Bacteria**: An imbalance in the gut microbiota can play a role in the development of IBS.

Inflammation:

• **Low-Grade Inflammation**: Some people with IBS may have low-grade inflammation in the gut.

<u>*Genetics*</u>:

• **Family History**: A genetic predisposition may increase the risk of developing IBS.

<u>**Management Strategies:**</u>

Understanding these triggers and causes can help in managing IBS. Strategies include:

- **Dietary Adjustments**: Following a low-FODMAP diet, avoiding trigger foods, and maintaining a balanced diet.

- **Stress Management**: Techniques like mindfulness, yoga, and cognitive-behavioral therapy (CBT) can help reduce stress-related symptoms.

- **Medications**: Depending on symptoms, medications such as antispasmodics, laxatives, or anti-diarrheal agents may be prescribed.

- **Probiotics**: These can help balance the gut microbiome.

- **Regular Exercise**: Physical activity can improve bowel function and reduce stress.

Working with a healthcare provider or a registered dietitian can help tailor a management plan to individual needs, improving quality of life for those with IBS.

Introduction To The Low FODMAP Diet & Benefits

The low-FODMAP diet is a scientifically proven approach to managing symptoms of Irritable Bowel Syndrome (IBS) and other functional gastrointestinal disorders.

This diet involves restricting foods that are high in certain types of carbohydrates known as FODMAPs, which can be difficult to digest for some people. Here's an introduction to the low-FODMAP diet and its benefits:

Fermentable:

- **Oligosaccharides** (e.g., fructans and galactans found in wheat, onions, garlic, legumes)
- **Disaccharides** (e.g., lactose found in dairy products)
- **Monosaccharides** (e.g., fructose found in apples, honey, high-fructose corn syrup)

- **Polyols** (e.g., sorbitol and mannitol found in some fruits, vegetables, and artificial sweeteners)

These carbohydrates can be poorly absorbed in the small intestine and fermented by gut bacteria, leading to symptoms like bloating, gas, abdominal pain, and diarrhea.

Phases of the Low-FODMAP Diet:

- **Elimination Phase**: All high-FODMAP foods are eliminated from the diet for 4-6 weeks to reduce symptoms.
- **Reintroduction Phase**: High-FODMAP foods are gradually reintroduced one at a time to identify specific triggers and tolerance levels.
- **Personalization Phase**: A long-term eating plan is developed based on the individual's specific FODMAP

tolerance, allowing for a more varied diet while managing symptoms.

Benefits of the Low-FODMAP Diet:

• **Symptom Relief**: The primary benefit is the significant reduction in IBS symptoms such as bloating, gas, abdominal pain, and irregular bowel movements. Studies show that around 70% of people with IBS experience symptom improvement on a low-FODMAP diet.

• **Improved Quality of Life**: By managing symptoms more effectively, individuals often experience an improved quality of life, including better sleep, increased energy levels, and enhanced mental well-being.

• **Personalized Nutrition**: The reintroduction phase helps identify specific food triggers, allowing for a more tailored and sustainable dietary approach. This personalization helps maintain long-term dietary diversity and nutritional balance.

• **Enhanced Gut Health**: While the initial elimination phase is restrictive, the overall process promotes better gut health by identifying and managing foods that cause discomfort, thus allowing for a more stable and comfortable digestive environment.

Practical Tips for the Low-FODMAP Diet:

- **Read Labels**: Be vigilant about food labels to identify high-FODMAP ingredients.
- **Meal Planning**: Plan meals and snacks to ensure a balanced intake of nutrients while avoiding high-FODMAP foods.
- **Hydration**: Drink plenty of water, especially when increasing fiber intake from low-FODMAP sources.

- **Support**: Consider working with a dietitian who specializes in the low-FODMAP diet for personalized guidance and support.

Common Low-FODMAP Foods:

- **Fruits**: Bananas, blueberries, strawberries, oranges, grapes
- **Vegetables**: Carrots, cucumbers, spinach, zucchini, bell peppers
- **Proteins**: Chicken, beef, fish, eggs, tofu
- **Grains**: Rice, oats, quinoa, gluten-free products
- **Dairy Alternatives**: Lactose-free milk, almond milk, coconut yogurt

The low-FODMAP diet is a valuable tool for individuals with IBS and other functional gastrointestinal disorders. By systematically eliminating and reintroducing high-FODMAP foods, it helps identify triggers and manage symptoms, leading to a better quality of life. For best results, it's recommended to undertake the diet under the guidance of a healthcare professional or a registered dietitian.

High FODMAP Foods To Avoid

If you're following a low-FODMAP diet to manage IBS or other gastrointestinal issues, it's crucial to avoid high-FODMAP foods that can trigger symptoms. Here are some common high-FODMAP foods to avoid across various categories:

- Fruits
- Apples
- Pears
- Watermelon
- Mangoes
- Cherries
- Plums
- Peaches
- Blackberries
- Vegetables
- Onions
- Garlic
- Cauliflower

- Broccoli

- Cabbage

- Asparagus

- Brussels sprouts

- Artichokes

- Mushrooms

- Grains and Cereals

- Wheat (including bread, pasta, cereals)

- Rye

- Barley

- Products containing high-fructose corn syrup

Dairy Products:

- Milk (cow, goat, sheep)

- Soft cheeses (e.g., ricotta, cottage cheese)

- Yogurt (regular and Greek)

- Ice cream

- Legumes and Pulses

- Lentils

- Chickpeas

- Beans (e.g., kidney beans, black beans)

- Soy products (except for tofu and tempeh)

Sweeteners and Sugar Alcohols:

- High-fructose corn syrup

- Honey

- Agave nectar

- Sorbitol

- Mannitol

- Xylitol

- Maltitol

<u>*Beverages:*</u>

- Fruit juices (from high-FODMAP fruits)

- Certain alcoholic beverages (e.g., rum, dessert wines)

- Soft drinks containing high-fructose corn syrup

<u>*Miscellaneous:*</u>

- Certain processed foods (check labels for high-FODMAP ingredients)

- Certain sauces and dressings (especially those with garlic and onions)

- Certain snack foods (like dried fruits and some energy bars)

<u>***Alternative Low-FODMAP Options:***</u>

<u>***Fruits:***</u>

- Bananas
- Blueberries
- Strawberries
- Oranges
- Kiwi
- Grapes
- Vegetables
- Carrots
- Spinach
- Zucchini
- Bell peppers
- Cucumbers
- Lettuce

<u>***Grains and Cereals:***</u>

- Rice (white, brown, basmati)
- Quinoa
- Oats

- Gluten-free bread and pasta

Dairy Alternatives:

- Lactose-free milk

- Almond milk

- Coconut milk

- Hard cheeses (e.g., cheddar, Parmesan)

- Lactose-free yogurt

Proteins:

- Chicken

- Beef

- Fish

- Eggs

- Tofu (firm, not silken)

- Tempeh

Tips for Following a Low-FODMAP Diet:

- **Meal Planning**: Plan meals and snacks ahead of time to ensure you have low-FODMAP options readily available.

- **Reading Labels**: Always check food labels for hidden high-FODMAP ingredients.

- **Cooking at Home**: Preparing meals at home allows you to control ingredients and avoid high-FODMAP foods.

- **Gradual Introduction**: If new to the diet, introduce low-FODMAP foods gradually to monitor your body's response.

By avoiding high-FODMAP foods and focusing on low-FODMAP alternatives, you can better manage IBS symptoms and improve your overall digestive health.

Low FODMAP Foods To Enjoy

Following a low-FODMAP diet involves focusing on foods that are less likely to trigger IBS symptoms. Here are some common low-FODMAP foods across various categories that you can enjoy:

Fruits:

- Bananas (ripe and firm)
- Blueberries
- Strawberries
- Oranges
- Kiwi
- Grapes
- Cantaloupe
- Pineapple
- Vegetables
- Carrots
- Spinach
- Zucchini
- Bell Peppers

- Cucumbers

- Lettuce (all varieties)

- Tomatoes

- Green Beans

- Eggplant

- Potatoes (white, red, sweet)

- Kale

Grains and Cereals:

- Rice (white, brown, basmati)

- Quinoa

- Oats (gluten-free)

- Polenta

- Cornflakes (without high-FODMAP ingredients)

- Gluten-Free Bread (check for FODMAP-friendly certification)

Dairy Alternatives:

- Lactose-Free Milk

- Almond Milk

- Coconut Milk

- Lactose-Free Yogurt

- Hard Cheeses (cheddar, Parmesan, Swiss)

- Butter (in moderation, as it contains very low lactose)

Proteins:

- Chicken

- Beef

- Fish (all types)

- Pork

- Eggs

- Firm Tofu

- Tempeh

Nuts and Seeds:

- Almonds (small quantities, up to 10 nuts)

- Peanuts

- Macadamia Nuts

- Pumpkin Seeds

- Sunflower Seeds

Sweeteners:

- Maple Syrup

- Table Sugar

- Stevia

- Sucrose

- Aspartame

Beverages:

- Water

- Lactose-Free Milk

- Almond Milk

- Green Tea

- Herbal Tea (peppermint, chamomile)

- Coffee (in moderation, with lactose-free or almond milk)

Herbs and Spices:

- Basil

- Chives

- Cilantro

- Parsley

- Rosemary

- Thyme

- Oregano

- Ginger

Snacks:

- Rice Cakes

- Popcorn

- Low-FODMAP Fruits (fresh or dried, such as strawberries or kiwi)

- Lactose-Free Yogurt with Berries

- Gluten-Free Crackers

Tips for Enjoying Low-FODMAP Foods:

- **Variety**: Ensure a balanced diet by including a variety of foods from all food groups.

- **Freshness**: Fresh, whole foods are often the best choices for a low-FODMAP diet.

- **Cooking Methods**: Grilling, steaming, roasting, and baking are good cooking methods that maintain the integrity of low-FODMAP foods.

- **Meal Planning**: Plan your meals and snacks in advance to ensure you have plenty of low-FODMAP options available.

- **Label Reading**: Always read labels on packaged foods to check for hidden high-FODMAP ingredients.

- **Portion Control**: Even low-FODMAP foods can cause symptoms if eaten in large quantities, so it's important to monitor portion sizes.

By incorporating these low-FODMAP foods into your diet, you can effectively manage IBS symptoms and enjoy a variety of tasty and nutritious meals.

CHAPTER THREE
Portion Sizes And Serving Suggestions

When following a low-FODMAP diet, portion sizes are crucial because even low-FODMAP foods can trigger symptoms if consumed in large quantities. Here are some guidelines on portion sizes and serving suggestions for various low-FODMAP foods:

Fruits:

- **Bananas**: 1 small banana (about 100g)
- **Blueberries**: 20 blueberries (about 28g)
- **Strawberries**: Up to 10 medium strawberries (about 140g)
- **Oranges**: 1 medium orange (about 130g)
- **Kiwi**: 2 small kiwis (about 150g)

- **Grapes**: 1 cup (about 150g)

- **Cantaloupe**: 1/2 cup (about 90g)

- **Pineapple**: 1 cup (about 140g)

Vegetables:

- **Carrots**: 1 medium carrot (about 50g)

- **Spinach**: 1 cup fresh (about 30g)

- **Zucchini**: 1/2 cup cooked (about 65g)

- **Bell Peppers**: 1/2 cup (about 50g)

- **Cucumbers**: 1/2 cup (about 52g)

- **Lettuce**: 1 cup (about 75g)

- **Tomatoes**: 1 small tomato (about 75g)

- **Green Beans**: 10 beans (about 75g)

- **Eggplant**: 3/4 cup (about 100g)

- **Potatoes**: 1 medium potato (about 150g)

Grains and Cereals:

- **Rice**: 1 cup cooked (about 190g)

- **Quinoa**: 1 cup cooked (about 185g)

- **Oats**: 1/2 cup rolled oats (about 40g)

- **Polenta**: 1 cup cooked (about 250g)

- **Cornflakes**: 1 cup (about 30g)

- **Gluten-Free Bread**: 1 slice (about 35g)

Dairy Alternatives:

- **Lactose-Free Milk**: 1 cup (about 250ml)

- **Almond Milk**: 1 cup (about 250ml)

- **Coconut Milk**: 1/2 cup (about 120ml)

- **Lactose-Free Yogurt**: 1 cup (about 170g)

- **Hard Cheeses**: 2 slices (about 40g)

- **Butter**: 1 pat (about 5g)

Proteins:

- **Chicken**: 1 serving (about 100g cooked)

- **Beef**: 1 serving (about 100g cooked)

- **Fish**: 1 serving (about 100g cooked)

- **Pork**: 1 serving (about 100g cooked)

- **Eggs**: 2 large eggs
- **Firm Tofu**: 1/2 cup (about 90g)
- **Tempeh**: 1/4 cup (about 50g)

Nuts and Seeds:

- **Almonds**: 10 nuts (about 12g)
- **Peanuts**: 32 nuts (about 28g)
- **Macadamia Nuts**: 10 nuts (about 15g)
- **Pumpkin Seeds**: 2 tablespoons (about 28g)
- **Sunflower Seeds**: 2 tablespoons (about 16g)

Sweeteners:

- **Maple Syrup**: 1 tablespoon (about 20g)
- **Table Sugar**: 1 tablespoon (about 13g)
- **Stevia**: According to package instructions
- **Sucrose**: 1 tablespoon (about 13g)

- **Aspartame**: According to package instructions

Beverages:

- **Water**: Unlimited
- **Lactose-Free Milk**: 1 cup (about 250ml)
- **Almond Milk**: 1 cup (about 250ml)
- **Green Tea**: 1 cup (about 250ml)
- **Herbal Tea**: 1 cup (about 250ml)
- **Coffee**: 1 cup (about 250ml)

Herbs and Spices:

- **Basil**: Unlimited
- **Chives**: Unlimited
- **Cilantro**: Unlimited
- **Parsley**: Unlimited
- **Rosemary**: Unlimited
- **Thyme**: Unlimited
- **Oregano**: Unlimited
- **Ginger**: Unlimited

- **Rice Cakes**: 2 cakes
- **Popcorn**: 3 cups (about 24g)
- **Low-FODMAP Fruits**: Appropriate portion sizes listed above
- **Lactose-Free Yogurt with Berries**: 1 cup yogurt with 20 blueberries
- **Gluten-Free Crackers**: 10 crackers (about 30g)

Tips for Portion Control:

- **Use Measuring Tools**: Utilize measuring cups, spoons, and a kitchen scale to ensure proper portion sizes.
- **Listen to Your Body**: Pay attention to how your body responds to different portion sizes and adjust accordingly.
- **Keep a Food Diary**: Track your food intake and symptoms to identify any potential triggers or portion-related issues.

- **Stay Informed**: Continually educate yourself on low-FODMAP foods and recommended portion sizes to maintain effective symptom management.

By following these portion sizes and serving suggestions, you can better manage IBS symptoms while enjoying a varied and nutritious diet.

Weekly Meal Planner

Creating a weekly meal planner for a low-FODMAP diet can help ensure you have a balanced, nutritious diet while managing IBS symptoms. Here's a sample meal plan, including breakfast, lunch, dinner, and snacks for each day.

Monday:

Breakfast:

- Low-FODMAP Smoothie: Spinach, banana, kiwi, almond milk

Lunch:

- Grilled Chicken Salad: Mixed greens, grilled chicken breast, bell peppers, carrots, cucumber, olive oil and lemon dressing

Dinner:

- Baked Salmon: Salmon fillet with lemon and herbs, served with steamed green beans and quinoa

Snacks:

- Lactose-free yogurt with strawberries
- Rice cakes with peanut butter

Tuesday:

Breakfast:

- Overnight Oats: Gluten-free oats, lactose-free milk, blueberries, chia seeds

Lunch:

- Turkey and Swiss Wrap: Gluten-free wrap with sliced turkey, Swiss cheese, lettuce, and mustard

Dinner:

- Stir-Fried Tofu: Firm tofu, zucchini, bell peppers, carrots, and bok choy stir-fried with tamari sauce, served with jasmine rice

Snacks:

- Orange slices
- Handful of almonds (10 nuts)

Wednesday

Breakfast:

- Scrambled Eggs: Eggs with spinach and chives, served with a slice of gluten-free toast

Lunch:

- Quinoa Salad: Quinoa, cherry tomatoes, cucumber, feta cheese, olives, and a lemon vinaigrette

Dinner:

- Beef Tacos: Ground beef, lettuce, tomatoes, lactose-free cheese, served in gluten-free taco shells

Snacks:

- Blueberries
- Carrot sticks with hummus

Thursday

Breakfast:

- Smoothie Bowl: Lactose-free yogurt, banana, pineapple, chia seeds, and a handful of blueberries

Lunch:

- Grilled Shrimp: Grilled shrimp on a bed of mixed greens with cucumber, tomatoes, and a lime vinaigrette

Dinner:

- Baked Chicken: Herb-marinated chicken breast, roasted sweet potatoes, and steamed broccoli

Snacks:

- Kiwi slices
- Popcorn (3 cups)

Friday

Breakfast:

- Greek Yogurt Parfait: Lactose-free Greek yogurt, strawberries, gluten-free granola

Lunch:

- Lentil Soup: Homemade low-FODMAP lentil soup with carrots, celery, and tomatoes

Dinner:

- Pork Tenderloin: Roasted pork tenderloin with mashed potatoes and sautéed spinach

Snacks:

- Orange slices
- Gluten-free crackers with cheddar cheese

Saturday

Breakfast:

- Omelette: Eggs with spinach, tomatoes, and a small amount of cheddar cheese

Lunch:

- Grilled Chicken Wrap: Gluten-free wrap with grilled chicken, lettuce, cucumber, and a low-FODMAP dressing

Dinner:

- Shrimp and Vegetable Skewers: Grilled shrimp, zucchini, bell peppers, and cherry tomatoes served with quinoa

Snacks:

- Grapes
- Rice cakes with almond butter

Sunday:

Breakfast:

- Pancakes: Gluten-free pancakes topped with strawberries and a drizzle of maple syrup

Lunch:

- Turkey Salad: Mixed greens with sliced turkey, avocado, cherry tomatoes, and a balsamic vinaigrette

Dinner:

- Baked Cod: Cod fillet with lemon and herbs, served with roasted carrots and green beans

Snacks:

- Kiwi slices
- Handful of macadamia nuts (10 nuts)

Tips for a Low-FODMAP Meal Planner:

- **Batch Cooking**: Prepare larger portions of certain meals (like soups and salads) and store leftovers for quick meals during the week.

- **Variety**: Include a wide range of fruits, vegetables, proteins, and grains to ensure nutritional balance.

- **Portion Control**: Stick to recommended portion sizes to avoid overconsumption of even low-FODMAP foods.

- **Preparation**: Pre-cut vegetables and pre-cook proteins (like grilled chicken or shrimp) to save time during the week.

- **Hydration**: Drink plenty of water throughout the day to aid digestion and overall health.

By following this meal planner, you can enjoy a variety of delicious and nutritious low-

FODMAP meals throughout the week, helping to manage IBS symptoms effectively.

CHAPTER FOUR
Cooking Tips And Techniques

Cooking low-FODMAP meals can be enjoyable and delicious with the right techniques and tips. Here are some practical cooking tips and techniques to help you prepare tasty and nutritious low-FODMAP dishes:

General Cooking Tips:

- **Batch Cooking**: Prepare large portions of meals like soups, stews, and casseroles, then freeze individual servings for quick and easy meals later.

- **Meal Prep**: Spend a few hours each week prepping ingredients (chopping vegetables, marinating proteins) to save time during busy weekdays.

- **Flavor Boosters**: Use fresh herbs, spices, lemon, lime, and infused oils to enhance flavor without relying on high-FODMAP ingredients like garlic and onions.

Cooking Techniques:

- **Roasting**: Roasting vegetables and proteins brings out natural flavors. Try roasting carrots, potatoes, and chicken with herbs and olive oil.

- **Grilling**: Grilling adds a smoky flavor to meats, fish, and vegetables. Marinate proteins in low-FODMAP herbs and spices for added taste.

- **Stir-Frying**: Quickly cook vegetables and proteins in a hot pan with a small amount of oil. Use tamari (gluten-free soy sauce) for seasoning.

- **Baking**: Baking is a versatile method for proteins, vegetables, and gluten-free baked goods. Use parchment paper to prevent sticking and reduce the need for excess oil.

- **Steaming**: Steaming preserves nutrients and flavors in vegetables. Use a steamer basket over boiling water and season with lemon and herbs.

- **Slow Cooking**: Slow cookers are perfect for making flavorful stews and soups. Combine low-FODMAP ingredients in the morning for a ready-to-eat dinner.

Ingredient Substitutions:

- **Garlic and Onion**: Use garlic-infused oil and the green parts of scallions or chives to mimic the flavor of garlic and onion without the FODMAPs.

- **Dairy**: Substitute regular milk with lactose-free milk, almond milk, or coconut milk. Use lactose-free yogurt and cheese.

- **Wheat**: Replace wheat-based products with gluten-free alternatives like rice, quinoa, and gluten-free bread and pasta.

Recipe Ideas:

- **Low-FODMAP Smoothie**: Blend spinach, banana, kiwi, and almond milk for a nutritious breakfast or snack.

- **Grilled Chicken Salad**: Combine mixed greens, grilled chicken breast, bell peppers, cucumbers, and a lemon-olive oil dressing.

- **Baked Salmon**: Season salmon fillets with lemon, dill, and olive oil, then bake and serve with steamed green beans and quinoa.

- **Stir-Fried Tofu and Vegetables**: Stir-fry firm tofu, zucchini, bell peppers, and carrots with tamari sauce and serve over jasmine rice.

- **Quinoa Salad**: Mix cooked quinoa with cherry tomatoes, cucumbers, feta cheese, olives, and a lemon vinaigrette.

- **Beef Tacos**: Use gluten-free taco shells filled with seasoned ground beef, lettuce, tomatoes, and lactose-free cheese.

- **Baked Chicken with Sweet Potatoes**: Roast herb-marinated chicken breast with sweet potato wedges and a side of sautéed spinach.

- **Shrimp Skewers**: Grill shrimp with zucchini, bell peppers, and cherry tomatoes on skewers, served with quinoa.

Tips for Baking:

- **Gluten-Free Flour Mixes**: Use gluten-free flour mixes for baking. Xanthan gum can help improve texture and binding in gluten-free baked goods.

- **Moisture Retention**: Gluten-free baking can be dry. Add ingredients like applesauce, mashed bananas, or yogurt to retain moisture.

- **Resting Dough**: Let gluten-free dough rest for 15-30 minutes before baking to improve texture.

- **Don't Overmix**: Overmixing gluten-free batters can lead to dense and heavy results. Mix just until combined.

<u>Storage and Reheating:</u>

- **Proper Storage**: Store leftovers in airtight containers in the refrigerator for up to 3-4 days or freeze for longer storage.

- **Reheating**: Reheat leftovers gently on the stove or in the microwave. Add a splash of water or broth to prevent drying out.

By using these cooking tips and techniques, you can create delicious low-FODMAP meals that help manage IBS symptoms while still enjoying a wide variety of flavors and textures.

Low FODMAP Breakfast Options Recipes

Here are three delicious low-FODMAP breakfast options along with their recipes:

1. Spinach and Tomato Omelette

Ingredients:

- 2 large eggs
- 1/4 cup spinach, chopped
- 1/4 cup cherry tomatoes, halved
- Salt and pepper, to taste
- Olive oil or lactose-free butter for cooking

Instructions:

- In a bowl, whisk the eggs together until well combined. Season with salt and pepper.
- Heat a non-stick skillet over medium heat and add a little olive oil or lactose-free butter.

- Add the chopped spinach and cherry tomatoes to the skillet and cook for 1-2 minutes until spinach wilts slightly.

- Pour the whisked eggs into the skillet, swirling to spread evenly.

- Cook the omelette for 2-3 minutes until the edges start to set. Use a spatula to gently lift the edges and allow the uncooked egg to flow underneath.

- Once the omelette is mostly set but still slightly runny on top, fold it in half and cook for another 1-2 minutes until cooked through.

- Slide the omelette onto a plate and serve hot.

2. Low-FODMAP Smoothie Bowl

Ingredients:

- 1/2 cup lactose-free yogurt
- 1/2 cup spinach

- 1/2 ripe banana

- 1/4 cup blueberries

- 1 tablespoon chia seeds (optional)

- Toppings: sliced strawberries, shredded coconut, gluten-free granola (check ingredients)

Instructions:

- In a blender, combine lactose-free yogurt, spinach, banana, blueberries, and chia seeds (if using). Blend until smooth.

- Pour the smoothie into a bowl.

- Arrange sliced strawberries, shredded coconut, and gluten-free granola on top as desired.

- Serve immediately and enjoy!

3. Overnight Chia Seed Pudding:

Ingredients:

- 1/4 cup chia seeds

- 1 cup lactose-free milk or almond milk

- 1/2 teaspoon vanilla extract

- 1 tablespoon maple syrup (optional, adjust to taste)

- Toppings: sliced kiwi, strawberries, blueberries, or any low-FODMAP fruits

Instructions:

- In a bowl or jar, combine chia seeds, lactose-free milk, vanilla extract, and maple syrup (if using). Stir well.
- Cover and refrigerate overnight or for at least 4 hours, stirring occasionally to prevent clumping.
- In the morning, stir the chia pudding well. If it's too thick, add a little more lactose-free milk to reach desired consistency.
- Top with sliced kiwi, strawberries, blueberries, or your favorite low-FODMAP fruits.
- Serve chilled and enjoy!

These breakfast options are not only low in FODMAPs but also nutritious and satisfying, making them perfect for managing IBS symptoms while starting your day right.

Smoothies And Juices

Smoothies and juices can be refreshing and nutritious options for those following a low-FODMAP diet. Here are some delicious recipes that are low in FODMAPs:

1. Berry Banana Smoothie:

Ingredients:

- 1/2 ripe banana
- 1/2 cup blueberries
- 1/2 cup strawberries
- 1 cup lactose-free milk or almond milk
- 1 tablespoon chia seeds (optional)
- Ice cubes (optional)

Instructions:

- Place all ingredients in a blender.
- Blend until smooth and creamy.
- Add ice cubes if desired for a colder consistency.

- Pour into a glass and serve immediately.

2. Tropical Green Smoothie:

Ingredients:

- 1/2 cup pineapple chunks
- 1/2 cup kiwi slices
- 1 cup spinach
- 1 tablespoon freshly grated ginger
- 1 cup coconut water
- Ice cubes (optional)

Instructions:

- Combine pineapple chunks, kiwi slices, spinach, ginger, and coconut water in a blender.
- Blend until smooth.
- Add ice cubes if desired and blend again until well combined.
- Pour into glasses and serve chilled.

<u>*3. Carrot Ginger Juice:*</u>

Ingredients:

- 3 medium carrots, peeled and chopped
- 1-inch piece of fresh ginger, peeled and chopped
- 1/2 cup fresh orange juice (about 1 large orange)
- 1/2 cup water
- Ice cubes (optional)

Instructions:

- Place chopped carrots, ginger, orange juice, and water in a blender.
- Blend until smooth.
- Strain the mixture through a fine mesh sieve to remove pulp, if desired.
- Serve over ice cubes if desired.

<u>*4. Citrus Mint Green Juice*</u>

Ingredients:

- 1 cucumber, peeled and chopped
- 1 cup spinach
- 1/2 cup fresh mint leaves
- Juice of 1 lime
- Juice of 1/2 lemon
- 1 cup water
- Ice cubes (optional)

Instructions:

- Combine cucumber, spinach, mint leaves, lime juice, lemon juice, and water in a blender.
- Blend until smooth.
- Strain the mixture through a fine mesh sieve to remove pulp, if desired.
- Serve over ice cubes if desired.

Tips for Low-FODMAP Smoothies and Juices:

• **Use Low-FODMAP Fruits**: Stick to fruits like berries, banana (in moderation), pineapple, kiwi (in moderation), and citrus fruits.

• **Avoid High-FODMAP Ingredients**: Steer clear of fruits like apples, pears, and mangoes, as well as high-FODMAP vegetables like cauliflower and mushrooms.

• **Choose Lactose-Free or Alternative Milks**: Opt for lactose-free milk, almond milk, or coconut milk instead of regular milk.

• **Add Protein and Healthy Fats**: Consider adding a scoop of low-FODMAP protein powder, chia seeds, or a tablespoon of nut butter for extra nutrition and satiety.

• **Experiment with Herbs and Spices**: Fresh herbs like mint or ginger can add flavor without adding FODMAPs.

Enjoy these refreshing smoothies and juices as part of your low-FODMAP diet to help

manage IBS symptoms while staying hydrated
and nourished.

Lunch Recipes

<u>***Light and Digestive-Friendly Meals recipes:***</u>

Here are three light and digestive-friendly meal recipes that are suitable for those following a low-FODMAP diet:

<u>***1. Grilled Lemon Herb Chicken with Quinoa Salad:***</u>

Ingredients for Grilled Lemon Herb Chicken:

- 2 boneless, skinless chicken breasts
- Juice of 1 lemon
- 1 tablespoon olive oil
- 1 teaspoon dried oregano
- Salt and pepper, to taste

Instructions for Grilled Lemon Herb Chicken:

- In a bowl, whisk together lemon juice, olive oil, dried oregano, salt, and pepper.

- Place chicken breasts in a shallow dish and pour the marinade over them. Ensure chicken is evenly coated. Marinate for at least 30 minutes.

- Preheat grill or grill pan over medium-high heat. Grill chicken for 6-7 minutes per side or until cooked through (internal temperature should reach 165°F or 74°C). Remove from grill and let rest for a few minutes before slicing.

Ingredients for Quinoa Salad:

- 1 cup cooked quinoa, cooled
- 1/2 cup cherry tomatoes, halved
- 1/2 cucumber, diced
- 1/4 cup chopped fresh parsley
- 2 tablespoons lemon juice
- 1 tablespoon olive oil
- Salt and pepper, to taste

Instructions for Quinoa Salad:

- In a large bowl, combine cooked quinoa, cherry tomatoes, cucumber, and parsley.
- In a small bowl, whisk together lemon juice, olive oil, salt, and pepper.
- Pour dressing over quinoa mixture and toss to combine.
- Serve grilled lemon herb chicken slices over quinoa salad.

2. Baked Salmon with Roasted Vegetables

Ingredients for Baked Salmon:

- 2 salmon fillets
- 1 tablespoon olive oil
- 1 tablespoon chopped fresh dill
- Juice of 1/2 lemon
- Salt and pepper, to taste

Instructions for Baked Salmon:

- Preheat oven to 400°F (200°C).
- Place salmon fillets on a baking sheet lined with parchment paper.
- Drizzle olive oil over salmon. Sprinkle with chopped dill, lemon juice, salt, and pepper.
- Bake for 12-15 minutes or until salmon flakes easily with a fork.

Ingredients for Roasted Vegetables:

- 1 zucchini, sliced
- 1 red bell pepper, sliced
- 1 yellow bell pepper, sliced

- 1 tablespoon olive oil

- Salt and pepper, to taste

Instructions for Roasted Vegetables:

- Preheat oven to 400°F (200°C).

- Toss sliced zucchini, red bell pepper, and yellow bell pepper with olive oil, salt, and pepper.

- Spread vegetables in a single layer on a baking sheet lined with parchment paper.

- Roast for 20-25 minutes or until vegetables are tender and slightly caramelized.

- Serve baked salmon with roasted vegetables.

Salads And Sandwiches Recipes

Here are some light and delicious salad and sandwich recipes suitable for a low-FODMAP diet:

1. Quinoa and Vegetable Salad

Ingredients:

- 1 cup cooked quinoa, cooled
- 1/2 cucumber, diced
- 1 cup cherry tomatoes, halved
- 1/4 cup chopped fresh parsley
- 1/4 cup chopped fresh mint
- Juice of 1 lemon
- 2 tablespoons olive oil
- Salt and pepper, to taste

Instructions:

- In a large bowl, combine cooked quinoa, cucumber, cherry tomatoes, parsley, and mint.
- In a small bowl, whisk together lemon juice, olive oil, salt, and pepper.
- Pour dressing over quinoa mixture and toss to combine.

- Serve chilled as a refreshing salad option.

2. Turkey and Swiss Lettuce Wraps

Ingredients:

- Large lettuce leaves (such as romaine or butter lettuce)
- Sliced turkey breast (check for no added high-FODMAP ingredients)
- Swiss cheese, sliced
- Sliced tomatoes
- Sliced cucumbers
- Mustard (check for low-FODMAP ingredients)
- Olive oil or mayonnaise (check for low-FODMAP ingredients)

Instructions:

- Lay out lettuce leaves flat on a clean surface.

- Spread a thin layer of mustard or olive oil/mayonnaise on each leaf.

- Layer with turkey slices, Swiss cheese, tomatoes, and cucumbers.

- Roll up each lettuce leaf tightly, securing with toothpicks if necessary.

- Serve immediately as a light and crunchy sandwich alternative.

3. Caprese Salad with Balsamic Glaze

Ingredients:

- Fresh mozzarella cheese, sliced
- Ripe tomatoes, sliced
- Fresh basil leaves
- Balsamic glaze (check for low-FODMAP ingredients)
- Olive oil
- Salt and pepper, to taste

Instructions:

- Arrange alternating slices of mozzarella cheese and tomatoes on a serving platter.
- Tuck fresh basil leaves between the cheese and tomatoes.
- Drizzle with balsamic glaze and olive oil.
- Season with salt and pepper to taste.
- Serve immediately as a light and flavorful salad option.

Tips for Low-FODMAP Salads and Sandwiches:

• **Choose Low-FODMAP Vegetables**: Opt for vegetables like lettuce, cucumber, tomatoes, bell peppers (red, yellow), and carrots.

• **Use Low-FODMAP Dressings**: Make or choose dressings with olive oil, lemon juice, vinegar (excluding apple cider vinegar), and low-FODMAP herbs like basil and parsley.

• **Check Cheese Ingredients**: Ensure cheeses are low in lactose or lactose-free.

• **Gluten-Free Options**: Use gluten-free bread or wraps for sandwiches if needed.

These recipes provide tasty options for light meals that are easy to prepare and suitable for managing IBS symptoms on a low-FODMAP diet.

Here are three delicious and soothing soup and broth recipes that are suitable for a low-FODMAP diet:

1. Carrot Ginger Soup:

Ingredients:

- 1 tablespoon olive oil
- 1 pound carrots, peeled and chopped
- 1-inch piece of fresh ginger, peeled and minced
- 4 cups low-FODMAP vegetable broth
- Salt and pepper, to taste
- Fresh chives, chopped (for garnish, optional)

Instructions:

- Heat olive oil in a large pot over medium heat.

- Add chopped carrots and minced ginger. Sauté for about 5 minutes until carrots start to soften.

- Pour in low-FODMAP vegetable broth. Bring to a boil, then reduce heat and simmer for 20-25 minutes until carrots are tender.

- Remove from heat and let cool slightly.

- Use an immersion blender to puree the soup until smooth. Alternatively, carefully transfer the soup in batches to a blender and blend until smooth.

- Season with salt and pepper to taste.

- Serve hot, garnished with chopped fresh chives if desired.

2. Chicken and Rice Soup

Ingredients:

- 1 tablespoon olive oil

- 2 boneless, skinless chicken breasts, cut into bite-sized pieces
- 1 carrot, diced
- 1 celery stalk, diced
- 1 cup cooked white rice
- 4 cups low-FODMAP chicken broth
- Salt and pepper, to taste
- Fresh parsley, chopped (for garnish, optional)

Instructions:

- Heat olive oil in a large pot over medium heat.
- Add diced chicken pieces and cook until browned and cooked through, about 5-7 minutes.
- Add diced carrot and celery to the pot. Sauté for another 3-4 minutes until vegetables start to soften.

- Pour in low-FODMAP chicken broth. Bring to a boil, then reduce heat and simmer for 15-20 minutes.

- Stir in cooked rice and simmer for another 5 minutes until heated through.

- Season with salt and pepper to taste.

- Serve hot, garnished with chopped fresh parsley if desired.

3. *Tomato Basil Soup*

Ingredients:

- 1 tablespoon olive oil
- 1 can (14 oz) diced tomatoes (check for no added high-FODMAP ingredients)
- 1 cup low-FODMAP vegetable broth
- 1/2 cup lactose-free cream or coconut cream
- 1/4 cup fresh basil leaves, chopped
- Salt and pepper, to taste

Instructions:

- Heat olive oil in a large pot over medium heat.
- Add diced tomatoes (including juice) to the pot. Cook for 5-7 minutes, stirring occasionally, until tomatoes start to break down.

- Pour in low-FODMAP vegetable broth. Bring to a boil, then reduce heat and simmer for 15 minutes.

- Remove from heat and let cool slightly.

- Use an immersion blender to puree the soup until smooth. Alternatively, carefully transfer the soup in batches to a blender and blend until smooth.

- Return soup to low heat. Stir in lactose-free cream or coconut cream and chopped fresh basil.

- Season with salt and pepper to taste.

- Serve hot, optionally garnished with additional basil leaves.

Tips for Low-FODMAP Soups and Broths:

- **Use Low-FODMAP Broths**: Choose broths labeled as low-FODMAP or make your own using low-FODMAP ingredients.

- **Check Canned Ingredients**: Be sure to check canned ingredients like tomatoes for added high-FODMAP ingredients such as onion or garlic.

- **Fresh Herbs and Spices**: Use fresh herbs like basil, parsley, and chives for flavor instead of high-FODMAP alternatives.

- **Serve with Caution**: Some individuals with IBS may find hot soups easier to digest than cold soups.

These soup and broth recipes are comforting, easy to prepare, and perfect for supporting digestive health while following a low-FODMAP diet.

Dinner Recipes

Hearty and Satisfying Dinners recipes

Here are three hearty and satisfying dinner recipes that are suitable for a low-FODMAP diet:

1. Lemon Herb Grilled Chicken with Quinoa Pilaf

Ingredients for Lemon Herb Grilled Chicken:

- 2 boneless, skinless chicken breasts
- Juice of 1 lemon
- 2 tablespoons olive oil
- 1 teaspoon dried oregano
- Salt and pepper, to taste

Instructions for Lemon Herb Grilled Chicken:

- In a bowl, whisk together lemon juice, olive oil, dried oregano, salt, and pepper.
- Place chicken breasts in a shallow dish and pour the marinade over them. Ensure chicken is evenly coated. Marinate for at least 30 minutes.

- Preheat grill or grill pan over medium-high heat. Grill chicken for 6-7 minutes per side or until cooked through (internal temperature should reach 165°F or 74°C). Remove from grill and let rest for a few minutes before slicing.

Ingredients for Quinoa Pilaf:

- 1 cup quinoa, rinsed and drained
- 2 cups low-FODMAP chicken or vegetable broth
- 1 tablespoon olive oil
- 1/4 cup pine nuts (optional)
- 1/4 cup chopped fresh parsley
- Salt and pepper, to taste

Instructions for Quinoa Pilaf:

- In a medium saucepan, heat olive oil over medium heat.

- Add rinsed quinoa and toast for 2-3 minutes until lightly golden and fragrant.

- Pour in low-FODMAP chicken or vegetable broth and bring to a boil.

- Reduce heat to low, cover, and simmer for 15-20 minutes or until quinoa is cooked and liquid is absorbed.

- Remove from heat and let sit for 5 minutes, then fluff with a fork.

- Stir in pine nuts (if using) and chopped fresh parsley. Season with salt and pepper to taste.

- Serve grilled lemon herb chicken slices over quinoa pilaf for a hearty and satisfying dinner.

<u>**2. Pan-Seared Salmon with Roasted Potatoes and Green Beans**</u>

Ingredients for Pan-Seared Salmon:

- 2 salmon fillets
- 1 tablespoon olive oil
- Salt and pepper, to taste
- Lemon wedges, for serving

Instructions for Pan-Seared Salmon:

- Pat salmon fillets dry with paper towels. Season both sides with salt and pepper.
- Heat olive oil in a large skillet over medium-high heat.
- Add salmon fillets, skin-side down, and cook for 4-5 minutes until skin is crispy and golden brown.
- Flip salmon fillets and cook for an additional 3-4 minutes, or until salmon

is cooked through and flakes easily with a fork.

- Remove from heat and squeeze lemon wedges over salmon before serving.

Ingredients for Roasted Potatoes and Green Beans:

- 1 pound baby potatoes, halved
- 1 pound green beans, trimmed
- 2 tablespoons olive oil
- Salt and pepper, to taste

Instructions for Roasted Potatoes and Green Beans:

- Preheat oven to 400°F (200°C).
- On a large baking sheet, toss halved baby potatoes and trimmed green beans with olive oil, salt, and pepper.
- Spread vegetables in a single layer on the baking sheet.

- Roast for 20-25 minutes, stirring halfway through, until potatoes are tender and green beans are lightly caramelized.

- Serve pan-seared salmon with roasted potatoes and green beans for a satisfying and nutritious dinner.

3. Quinoa Stuffed Bell Peppers

Ingredients:

- 4 large bell peppers, tops cut off and seeds removed

- 1 cup quinoa, rinsed and drained

- 2 cups low-FODMAP vegetable broth

- 1 tablespoon olive oil

- 1/2 cup diced tomatoes (canned, check for low-FODMAP ingredients)

- 1/2 cup chopped spinach

- 1/4 cup chopped fresh parsley

- Salt and pepper, to taste

- Grated lactose-free cheese (optional, for topping)

Instructions:

- Preheat oven to 375°F (190°C).

- In a medium saucepan, heat olive oil over medium heat.

- Add rinsed quinoa and toast for 2-3 minutes until lightly golden and fragrant.

- Pour in low-FODMAP vegetable broth and bring to a boil.

- Reduce heat to low, cover, and simmer for 15-20 minutes or until quinoa is cooked and liquid is absorbed.

- Remove from heat and let sit for 5 minutes, then fluff with a fork.

- Stir in diced tomatoes, chopped spinach, and chopped fresh parsley. Season with salt and pepper to taste.

- Spoon quinoa mixture evenly into prepared bell peppers, packing lightly.

- Place stuffed bell peppers upright in a baking dish. If desired, top with grated lactose-free cheese.

- Cover with foil and bake for 25-30 minutes, until bell peppers are tender.

- Serve quinoa stuffed bell peppers hot as a hearty and satisfying vegetarian dinner option.

These dinner recipes are flavorful, nutritious, and designed to be low in FODMAPs to support digestive health. Enjoy these hearty meals as part of your low-FODMAP diet plan.

Here are three comforting and easy one-pot and slow cooker meals that are suitable for a low-FODMAP diet:

1. One-Pot Chicken and Vegetable Stir-Fry

Ingredients:

- 1 tablespoon garlic-infused olive oil
- 2 boneless, skinless chicken breasts, cut into bite-sized pieces
- 1 red bell pepper, sliced
- 1 zucchini, sliced
- 1 cup carrots, sliced
- 1 cup green beans, trimmed
- 1/4 cup low-sodium tamari sauce (gluten-free soy sauce)
- 1 tablespoon rice vinegar
- 1 tablespoon maple syrup (or other low-FODMAP sweetener)
- Cooked rice or quinoa, for serving

Instructions:

- In a large skillet or pot, heat garlic-infused olive oil over medium-high heat.

- Add chicken breast pieces and cook until browned and cooked through, about 5-7 minutes.

- Add sliced red bell pepper, zucchini, carrots, and green beans to the skillet. Stir-fry for another 5 minutes until vegetables are tender-crisp.

- In a small bowl, whisk together tamari sauce, rice vinegar, and maple syrup. Pour over chicken and vegetables in the skillet.

- Stir to coat everything evenly with the sauce. Cook for an additional 2-3 minutes until heated through.

- Serve hot over cooked rice or quinoa.

2. Slow Cooker Beef Stew

Ingredients:

- 1.5 pounds stewing beef, cut into cubes
- 4 cups low-FODMAP beef broth
- 1 cup carrots, sliced
- 1 cup potatoes, diced (check for low-FODMAP options)
- 1 cup celery, sliced
- 1 cup green beans, trimmed
- 1 tablespoon tomato paste
- 1 teaspoon dried thyme
- Salt and pepper, to taste

Instructions:

- In a slow cooker, combine stewing beef, low-FODMAP beef broth, sliced carrots, diced potatoes, sliced celery, trimmed green beans, tomato paste, dried thyme, salt, and pepper.
- Stir to combine all ingredients.

- Cover and cook on low for 6-8 hours or on high for 3-4 hours, until beef and vegetables are tender.
- Taste and adjust seasoning if needed before serving.
- Serve hot, optionally garnished with fresh parsley.

3. One-Pot Mediterranean Quinoa

Ingredients:

- 1 tablespoon olive oil
- 1 pound boneless, skinless chicken thighs, cut into bite-sized pieces
- 1 cup quinoa, rinsed and drained
- 2 cups low-FODMAP chicken broth
- 1 cup cherry tomatoes, halved
- 1/2 cup Kalamata olives, pitted and sliced
- 1/4 cup chopped fresh parsley
- Juice of 1 lemon
- Salt and pepper, to taste

Instructions:

- In a large pot or Dutch oven, heat olive oil over medium-high heat.
- Add chicken thigh pieces and cook until browned and cooked through, about 6-8 minutes.
- Add rinsed and drained quinoa to the pot. Stir for 1-2 minutes to toast the quinoa.
- Pour in low-FODMAP chicken broth and bring to a boil.
- Reduce heat to low, cover, and simmer for 15-20 minutes or until quinoa is cooked and liquid is absorbed.
- Stir in halved cherry tomatoes, sliced Kalamata olives, chopped fresh parsley, and lemon juice.
- Season with salt and pepper to taste.
- Serve hot, optionally garnished with additional parsley.

These one-pot and slow cooker meals are hearty, flavorful, and perfect for making low-FODMAP cooking easy and convenient. Enjoy these comforting dishes as part of your balanced diet plan.

Vegetarian And Vegan Options Recipes

Here are three delicious vegetarian and vegan options that are suitable for a low-FODMAP diet:

1. Quinoa Stuffed Bell Peppers

Ingredients:

- 4 large bell peppers, tops cut off and seeds removed
- 1 cup quinoa, rinsed and drained
- 2 cups low-FODMAP vegetable broth
- 1 tablespoon olive oil
- 1/2 cup diced tomatoes (canned, check for low-FODMAP ingredients)
- 1/2 cup chopped spinach
- 1/4 cup chopped fresh parsley
- Salt and pepper, to taste
- Grated lactose-free cheese (optional, for topping)

Instructions:

- Preheat oven to 375°F (190°C).

- In a medium saucepan, heat olive oil over medium heat.

- Add rinsed quinoa and toast for 2-3 minutes until lightly golden and fragrant.

- Pour in low-FODMAP vegetable broth and bring to a boil.

- Reduce heat to low, cover, and simmer for 15-20 minutes or until quinoa is cooked and liquid is absorbed.

- Remove from heat and let sit for 5 minutes, then fluff with a fork.

- Stir in diced tomatoes, chopped spinach, and chopped fresh parsley. Season with salt and pepper to taste.

- Spoon quinoa mixture evenly into prepared bell peppers, packing lightly.

- Place stuffed bell peppers upright in a baking dish. If desired, top with grated lactose-free cheese.

- Cover with foil and bake for 25-30 minutes, until bell peppers are tender.
- Serve quinoa stuffed bell peppers hot as a hearty and satisfying vegetarian dinner option.

2. Tofu Stir-Fry with Bok Choy

Ingredients:

- 1 tablespoon garlic-infused olive oil
- 1 block (14 oz) extra firm tofu, drained and cut into cubes
- 1 red bell pepper, sliced
- 1 zucchini, sliced
- 1 cup bok choy, chopped
- 2 tablespoons low-sodium tamari sauce (gluten-free soy sauce)
- 1 tablespoon rice vinegar
- 1 tablespoon maple syrup (or other low-FODMAP sweetener)
- Cooked rice or quinoa, for serving

Instructions:

- In a large skillet or wok, heat garlic-infused olive oil over medium-high heat.

- Add cubed tofu and cook until lightly browned on all sides, about 5-7 minutes.

- Add sliced red bell pepper, zucchini, and chopped bok choy to the skillet. Stir-fry for another 5 minutes until vegetables are tender-crisp.

- In a small bowl, whisk together tamari sauce, rice vinegar, and maple syrup. Pour over tofu and vegetables in the skillet.

- Stir to coat everything evenly with the sauce. Cook for an additional 2-3 minutes until heated through.

- Serve hot over cooked rice or quinoa.

3. Lentil and Spinach Curry

Ingredients:

- 1 tablespoon olive oil
- 1 cup dried red lentils, rinsed
- 1 can (14 oz) diced tomatoes (check for low-FODMAP ingredients)
- 1 can (14 oz) coconut milk (check for low-FODMAP ingredients)
- 2 cups baby spinach
- 1 tablespoon curry powder
- 1/2 teaspoon ground turmeric
- Salt and pepper, to taste
- Cooked rice, for serving

Instructions:

- In a large pot or Dutch oven, heat olive oil over medium heat.
- Add rinsed red lentils and sauté for 1-2 minutes.
- Stir in diced tomatoes (including juice), coconut milk, curry powder, and ground turmeric.

- Bring to a boil, then reduce heat to low and simmer for 20-25 minutes, stirring occasionally, until lentils are tender and curry has thickened.
- Stir in baby spinach and cook for another 2-3 minutes until spinach is wilted.
- Season with salt and pepper to taste.
- Serve hot over cooked rice.

These vegetarian and vegan options are flavorful, nutritious, and designed to be low in FODMAPs to support digestive health. Enjoy these delicious dishes as part of your balanced diet plan.

Snacks And Desserts

Healthy and Portable Snacks recipes

Here are three healthy and portable snack recipes that are suitable for a low-FODMAP diet:

1. Rice Cake with Almond Butter and Banana Slices

Ingredients:

- Rice cakes (check for low-FODMAP ingredients)
- Almond butter (or other low-FODMAP nut or seed butter)
- 1 banana, sliced

Instructions:

- Spread almond butter on top of a rice cake.
- Top with banana slices.
- Enjoy immediately or wrap in foil or a small container for a portable snack.

2. Trail Mix with Nuts and Seeds

Ingredients:

- 1/4 cup almonds, unsalted
- 1/4 cup pumpkin seeds (pepitas)

- 1/4 cup sunflower seeds

- 1/4 cup dried cranberries (check for low-FODMAP ingredients)

Instructions:

- Combine almonds, pumpkin seeds, sunflower seeds, and dried cranberries in a small bowl.
- Mix well.
- Portion into small resealable bags or containers for easy grab-and-go snacks.

3. Cucumber Slices with Hummus

Ingredients:

- 1 cucumber, sliced
- Low-FODMAP hummus (store-bought or homemade*)

Instructions:

- Slice cucumber into rounds.
- Serve with a side of low-FODMAP hummus for dipping.

- Pack in a small container for a refreshing and crunchy snack.

Low-FODMAP Hummus Recipe:

- 1 can (15 oz) chickpeas, drained and rinsed
- 1/4 cup tahini (sesame seed paste)
- Juice of 1 lemon
- 2 tablespoons garlic-infused olive oil
- Salt and pepper, to taste

Instructions for Hummus:

- In a food processor, combine chickpeas, tahini, lemon juice, and garlic-infused olive oil.
- Blend until smooth, scraping down the sides as needed.
- Season with salt and pepper to taste.
- Store in an airtight container in the refrigerator for up to one week.

These snack ideas are not only delicious but also convenient for taking on the go. They provide a balance of protein, healthy fats, and carbohydrates while being gentle on the digestive system for those following a low-FODMAP diet. Enjoy these snacks as part of your daily routine to keep energy levels up and hunger at bay.

Low FODMAP Desserts Recipes

Here are three delicious low-FODMAP dessert recipes that you can enjoy:

1. Raspberry Coconut Chia Pudding

Ingredients:

- 1/4 cup chia seeds
- 1 cup unsweetened coconut milk (check for low-FODMAP ingredients)
- 1 tablespoon maple syrup (or other low-FODMAP sweetener)
- 1/2 teaspoon vanilla extract
- 1/2 cup fresh raspberries

Instructions:

- In a bowl, combine chia seeds, unsweetened coconut milk, maple syrup, and vanilla extract.
- Stir well to combine.

- Cover and refrigerate for at least 2 hours or overnight, until the mixture thickens and forms a pudding-like consistency.

- Stir again before serving to ensure even texture.

- Top with fresh raspberries before serving.

2. Almond Flour Chocolate Chip Cookies

Ingredients:

- 1 cup almond flour
- 1/4 cup maple syrup (or other low-FODMAP sweetener)
- 1/4 cup coconut oil, melted
- 1/2 teaspoon vanilla extract
- 1/4 teaspoon baking soda
- Pinch of salt
- 1/3 cup dairy-free chocolate chips (check for low-FODMAP ingredients)

Instructions:

- Preheat oven to 350°F (175°C). Line a baking sheet with parchment paper.
- In a bowl, combine almond flour, maple syrup, melted coconut oil, vanilla extract, baking soda, and salt. Mix until well combined.
- Fold in dairy-free chocolate chips.
- Scoop tablespoons of dough and roll into balls. Place them on the prepared baking sheet, spacing them about 2 inches apart.
- Flatten each ball slightly with the palm of your hand.
- Bake for 10-12 minutes, until cookies are golden brown around the edges.
- Remove from oven and let cool on the baking sheet for 5 minutes before transferring to a wire rack to cool completely.

3. Pineapple Coconut Nice Cream

Ingredients:

- 2 cups frozen pineapple chunks
- 1 can (14 oz) coconut milk (check for low-FODMAP ingredients)
- 1 tablespoon maple syrup (or other low-FODMAP sweetener)
- 1/2 teaspoon vanilla extract

Instructions:

- In a blender or food processor, combine frozen pineapple chunks, coconut milk, maple syrup, and vanilla extract.

- Blend until smooth and creamy, scraping down the sides as needed.

- If needed, add a little more coconut milk to achieve the desired consistency.

- Serve immediately as soft-serve ice cream, or transfer to a container and freeze for 1-2 hours for a firmer texture.

- Scoop into bowls and enjoy!

These low-FODMAP dessert recipes are delicious treats that can satisfy your sweet cravings while being gentle on the digestive system. Enjoy them as part of a balanced diet, and feel free to adjust ingredients based on your preferences and tolerance levels.

Beverages And Smoothies Snacks Recipes

Here are three refreshing and low-FODMAP beverage and smoothie recipes that make for excellent snacks:

1. Tropical Green Smoothie

Ingredients:

- 1 cup fresh spinach
- 1/2 cup frozen pineapple chunks
- 1/2 cup frozen mango chunks
- 1/2 ripe banana (optional, adjust according to tolerance)
- 1 cup unsweetened almond milk (check for low-FODMAP ingredients)
- Juice of 1/2 lime
- Ice cubes (optional, for a colder smoothie)

Instructions:

- Place spinach, frozen pineapple chunks, frozen mango chunks, ripe banana (if using), almond milk, and lime juice in a blender.

- Blend until smooth and creamy.

- If desired, add ice cubes and blend again until smooth.

- Pour into a glass and serve immediately.

2. Iced Mint Green Tea

Ingredients:

- 2 cups water
- 2 green tea bags
- 1/4 cup fresh mint leaves, plus extra for garnish
- Ice cubes
- Optional: maple syrup or other low-FODMAP sweetener, to taste

Instructions:

- Bring water to a boil in a small saucepan.
- Remove from heat and add green tea bags and fresh mint leaves.
- Steep for 3-5 minutes, depending on desired strength.
- Remove tea bags and strain out mint leaves.

- Stir in maple syrup or other low-FODMAP sweetener if using.

- Allow tea to cool to room temperature, then transfer to the refrigerator to chill.

- Serve over ice cubes, garnished with fresh mint leaves.

3. Raspberry Coconut Water Refresher

Ingredients:

- 1 cup fresh raspberries

- 2 cups coconut water (check for low-FODMAP ingredients)

- Juice of 1 lime

- Ice cubes

- Fresh mint leaves, for garnish

Instructions:

- In a blender, combine fresh raspberries, coconut water, and lime juice.

- Blend until smooth.

- Strain the mixture through a fine mesh sieve to remove seeds, if desired.

- Pour over ice cubes in glasses.

- Garnish with fresh mint leaves.

- Serve immediately.

These beverage and smoothie recipes are not only delicious but also refreshing and suitable for a low-FODMAP diet. They provide hydration and nutrients without triggering digestive issues, making them perfect for a quick snack or a light refreshment throughout the day.

CHAPTER FIVE
Navigating Restaurant Menus

Navigating restaurant menus while following a low-FODMAP diet can be challenging but manageable with a few strategies. Here are some tips to help you make informed choices:

• Before going to a restaurant, check if they have their menu available online. This allows you to review options and plan your meal in advance.

• Opt for dishes that are simply grilled, roasted, or steamed. These cooking methods are less likely to include high-FODMAP ingredients like garlic or onion.

• Many sauces, dressings, and condiments contain high-FODMAP ingredients. Ask for sauces on the side or opt for olive oil, vinegar, or lemon juice as alternatives.

• Inform your server about your dietary restrictions and ask questions about how dishes are prepared. They can often provide insights and help you make suitable choices.

• Look for dishes centered around grilled meats, fish, or tofu, paired with low-

FODMAP vegetables such as carrots, bell peppers, or spinach.

• Salads can be tricky due to dressings and raw vegetables. Ask for dressings on the side or inquire about options with low-FODMAP ingredients.

• Don't hesitate to ask for modifications to dishes. For example, request to omit onions or garlic from stir-fries or substitute a side dish for something low-FODMAP.

• Side dishes like steamed rice, baked potatoes (without toppings), or steamed vegetables are generally safer options. Confirm how they are prepared to avoid hidden FODMAPs.

• Stick to safe beverages such as water, herbal teas, or coffee (without milk if lactose intolerant). Avoid sugary drinks and cocktails with unknown ingredients.

• Large portions can be overwhelming and may contain more FODMAPs. Consider appetizers or smaller portions if available.

• Desserts often contain high-FODMAP ingredients like wheat, dairy, or excess sugars. Inquire about suitable options or consider enjoying a low-FODMAP dessert at home.

• If unsure about options, having a small snack like nuts, rice cakes, or a piece of fruit you know is safe can prevent hunger while you decide.

By using these tips and communicating clearly with restaurant staff, you can navigate restaurant menus more confidently while sticking to your low-FODMAP diet. It's also helpful to stay flexible and patient, as some restaurants may be willing to accommodate special dietary needs with advance notice.

Managing Stress And IBS

Managing stress is crucial for individuals with IBS (Irritable Bowel Syndrome) because stress can exacerbate symptoms such as abdominal pain, bloating, and changes in bowel habits. Here are several strategies to help manage stress effectively:

1. Identify Stress Triggers:

• Keep a journal to identify situations, events, or people that trigger stress. Understanding these triggers can help you develop strategies to cope with them.

2. *Practice Relaxation Techniques:*

• **Deep Breathing:** Practice deep breathing exercises to calm your mind and body. Focus on slow, deep breaths in through your nose and out through your mouth.

• **Progressive Muscle Relaxation:** Tense and then relax different muscle groups in your body, starting from your toes up to your head. This technique helps release physical tension.

• **Mindfulness Meditation:** Practice mindfulness techniques to stay present and reduce anxiety. Apps like Headspace or Calm can guide you through meditation sessions.

3. Regular Physical Activity:

• Engage in regular exercise such as walking, jogging, yoga, or swimming. Exercise releases endorphins, which can improve mood and reduce stress levels.

4. Establish a Routine:

• Create a daily routine that includes regular sleep patterns, balanced meals, and time for relaxation. A consistent routine can provide a sense of stability and reduce stress.

5. Healthy Diet:

• Follow a well-balanced, low-FODMAP diet as recommended by your healthcare provider or dietitian. Avoid triggers such as caffeine, alcohol, and high-fat or spicy foods that can exacerbate IBS symptoms.

6. Get Adequate Sleep:

• Prioritize getting enough sleep each night (7-9 hours for most adults). Good sleep hygiene practices, such as establishing a bedtime routine and creating a comfortable sleep environment, can improve sleep quality.

7. Social Support:

• Maintain connections with supportive friends, family members, or support groups. Talking about your feelings and experiences with others can help reduce stress and provide emotional support.

8. Limit Stressful Situations:

• When possible, avoid or minimize exposure to stressful situations. Learn to say no to additional responsibilities or commitments if they contribute to stress.

9. Seek Professional Help:

• Consider speaking with a therapist or counselor who specializes in stress management or cognitive-behavioral therapy (CBT). Therapy can provide strategies to cope with stress more effectively.

10. Mind-Body Practices:

• Explore practices such as yoga, tai chi, or acupuncture, which can promote relaxation, improve mindfulness, and reduce stress levels.

11. Take Breaks and Practice Self-Care:

• Incorporate regular breaks throughout your day to rest and recharge. Engage in activities you enjoy, such as reading, listening to music, or spending time in nature.

12. Stay Informed and Educated:

• Educate yourself about IBS and its management strategies. Understanding your condition can empower you to make informed decisions and take control of your health.

By incorporating these stress management techniques into your daily routine, you can help reduce stress levels and potentially improve symptoms associated with IBS. It's essential to find a combination of strategies that work best for you and to practice them consistently for long-term benefit. If stress management techniques alone are not sufficient, consider discussing additional options with your healthcare provider.

CHAPTER SIX
Exercise And Physical Activity

Exercise and physical activity can be beneficial for managing IBS (Irritable Bowel Syndrome) symptoms, although it's essential to approach it carefully, as intense or high-impact exercise might exacerbate symptoms for some individuals. Here are some guidelines and considerations for incorporating exercise into your routine with IBS:

1. Choose Gentle Exercises:

• **Walking:** Brisk walking is a low-impact exercise that can help improve digestion and reduce stress.

• **Yoga:** Gentle yoga poses and stretches can promote relaxation, improve flexibility, and aid digestion.

• **Swimming:** Swimming or water aerobics provide a low-impact workout that is gentle on the joints and may help alleviate stress.

2. *Moderation is Key:*

• Start with short sessions of exercise and gradually increase intensity and duration as tolerated. Overexertion can trigger symptoms, so listen to your body and pace yourself.

3. *Timing of Exercise:*

• Some individuals find it beneficial to exercise in the morning to help regulate bowel movements. Experiment with different times of the day to see what works best for you.

4. Stay Hydrated:

• Drink plenty of water before, during, and after exercise to stay hydrated. Dehydration can exacerbate symptoms such as constipation.

5. Mind-Body Connection:

• Incorporate mindfulness techniques such as deep breathing or meditation before or after exercise to help reduce stress and improve overall well-being.

6. Avoid Trigger Foods Before Exercise:

• If certain foods trigger your symptoms, avoid consuming them before exercising to prevent discomfort during your workout.

7. Consult with a Healthcare Provider:

• If you have concerns about starting an exercise program or if your symptoms worsen with physical activity, consult with your healthcare provider or a physical therapist. They can provide personalized recommendations based on your health status and symptoms.

8. Listen to Your Body:

• If you experience abdominal pain, bloating, or other symptoms during exercise, stop and rest. It may be helpful to keep a journal to track how different types and intensities of exercise affect your symptoms.

9. Combine with Stress Management:

• Incorporate stress-reducing activities such as yoga, tai chi, or meditation into your exercise routine to help manage stress, which can contribute to IBS symptoms.

10. Consistency is Key:

• Aim for consistency in your exercise routine. Regular physical activity can help improve overall health, manage stress, and potentially alleviate some IBS symptoms over time.

By incorporating gentle and mindful exercises into your routine, you can potentially improve your overall well-being and manage IBS symptoms more effectively. It's important to find activities that you enjoy and that work well with your individual needs and limitations.

Long-Term Management And Support

Long-term management of IBS (Irritable Bowel Syndrome) involves a holistic approach that focuses on symptom management, lifestyle modifications, and ongoing support. Here are key strategies for long-term management and support:

1. Medical Guidance:

• **Consult with Healthcare Providers:** Work closely with a gastroenterologist or healthcare provider specializing in digestive health. They can diagnose IBS, rule out other conditions, and develop a personalized treatment plan.

• **Medication Management:** Depending on your symptoms, your doctor may prescribe medications such as antispasmodics, laxatives, or medications targeting specific symptoms like diarrhea or constipation.

- **Regular Follow-ups:** Schedule regular check-ups with your healthcare provider to monitor symptoms, adjust treatment if necessary, and address any concerns.

2. Dietary Management:

- **Low-FODMAP Diet:** Consider following a low-FODMAP diet under the guidance of a registered dietitian. This diet can help identify and reduce triggers that exacerbate symptoms.

- **Balanced Nutrition:** Ensure you are getting adequate fiber, fluids, and nutrients in your diet. Avoiding large meals and eating smaller, more frequent meals can also be beneficial.

- **Food Journaling:** Keep a food diary to track your diet and symptoms. This can help identify patterns and determine which foods may be contributing to your symptoms.

3. Lifestyle Modifications:

- **Stress Management:** Practice stress-reduction techniques such as meditation, deep breathing, yoga, or mindfulness. Chronic stress can worsen IBS symptoms.

- **Regular Exercise:** Engage in regular physical activity, such as walking, swimming, or yoga, to improve digestion, reduce stress, and promote overall well-being.

- **Adequate Sleep:** Prioritize good sleep hygiene and aim for 7-9 hours of quality sleep each night. Poor sleep can exacerbate symptoms of IBS.

4. Psychological Support:

- **Cognitive Behavioral Therapy (CBT):** Consider therapy with a psychologist or counselor trained in CBT. CBT can help manage stress, anxiety, and depression, which are common in individuals with IBS.

• **Support Groups:** Joining support groups or online forums can provide emotional support, shared experiences, and coping strategies from others living with IBS.

5. *Education and Self-Care:*

• **Learn About IBS:** Educate yourself about IBS, including its symptoms, triggers, and treatment options. Understanding your condition can empower you to make informed decisions.

• **Self-Care Practices:** Incorporate self-care activities into your daily routine, such as relaxation techniques, hobbies, and activities that promote mental and emotional well-being.

6. *Alternative Therapies:*

• **Acupuncture or Hypnotherapy:** Some individuals find relief from IBS symptoms through acupuncture or hypnotherapy. Discuss these options with your healthcare provider to see if they may be appropriate for you.

7. *Regular Monitoring and Adjustment:*

• **Track Symptoms:** Keep track of your symptoms, triggers, and response to treatments. This information can guide adjustments to your management plan.

• **Adapt as Needed:** Be prepared to make adjustments to your diet, lifestyle, and treatment plan based on changes in symptoms or new research findings.

8. *Long-Term Outlook:*

• **Stay Positive:** While managing IBS can be challenging, many individuals find significant relief with a combination of strategies tailored to their needs. Stay patient and proactive in managing your health.

With the help of your healthcare team and these tactics, you can create a long-term plan to manage irritable bowel syndrome (IBS) that will enhance your quality of life and reduce the frequency and severity of symptom flare-ups. Since IBS affects people differently, it may take some trial and error to discover a solution that works for you.

Summary

Irritable Bowel Syndrome (IBS) management, in conclusion, calls for an all-encompassing, individual strategy that takes into account the psychological and physiological components of the illness. Patients with irritable bowel syndrome (IBS) can greatly benefit from medical treatment, dietary management, behavioural changes, and emotional support in order to alleviate symptoms and enhance overall well-being.

For a precise diagnosis and the creation of a personalized treatment plan, medical advice from a healthcare professional focusing on digestive health is essential. Medication for gastrointestinal issues including gas, bloating, diarrhea, or constipation may be part of this.

Treatment can be adjusted according to your reaction and evolving symptoms when you have frequent checkups with your doctor. The low-FODMAP diet is frequently suggested as a means to identify and remove items that trigger symptoms, and dietary control plays a crucial role in this process.

To maintain a healthy diet and avoid foods that make symptoms worse, it is recommended to consult a qualified dietitian. Keeping a food journal can help people see connections between what they eat and how they feel, which in turn can help them make better dietary decisions. Making changes to one's lifestyle, such as exercising regularly and practicing stress management techniques (such as yoga, meditation, or mindfulness), can improve one's health in general and make irritable bowel syndrome (IBS) symptoms less severe.

Getting enough sleep and sticking to a schedule every day also help with intestinal health.

Anxiety, despair, and stress are common symptoms of irritable bowel syndrome (IBS), but they can be better managed with psychological support from therapies like cognitive behavioral therapy (CBT) or by joining a support group.

In order to help people cope with their symptoms, these interventions offer emotional support and coping mechanisms.

Essential components of long-term management include education about irritable bowel syndrome (IBS) and self-care routines. People can better take charge of their health and make educated decisions regarding treatment and lifestyle changes when they have a good grasp of the illness. Taking time for oneself to engage in pleasurable pursuits, such as hobbies, is an important part of maintaining good health.

Managing irritable bowel syndrome (IBS) is an ongoing process that calls for perseverance, flexibility, and understanding of each person's unique needs and reactions. Better symptom control, quality of life, and general wellness can be achieved by incorporating these approaches into everyday living and maintaining open communication with healthcare practitioners for those with IBS.

THE END